COPYRIGHT © 2024
ALL RIGHTS RESERVED.
NO PORTION OF THIS BOOK MAY BE REPRODUCED IN ANY FORM
WITHOUT WRITTEN PERMISSION FROM THE PUBLISHER OR AUTHOR,
EXCEPT AS PERMITTED BY U.S. COPYRIGHT LAW.

Dear Mama, This One's for You

Hey you, the one running on caffeine and cuddles, balancing a million things at once, and somehow still managing to keep everyone alive—**this book is for you.**

Motherhood isn't about having it all together (spoiler: no one does). It's about love, resilience, and showing up, even on the days when your patience is running on fumes and your idea of self-care is eating a snack without sharing.

In between the never-ending snack requests, the spontaneous toddler meltdowns, and the mountain of laundry that never seems to shrink, there is magic—hidden in the tiny hands reaching for yours, the sleepy whispers of "I love you, mommy", and the uncontrollable giggles over absolutely nothing.

This book is like a chat with your best mom friend—full of wisdom, encouragement, and laugh-out-loud moments to remind you that you are doing better than you think. It's here to lift you up when the mom guilt creeps in, to reassure you that you are enough, and to celebrate the beautifully messy, hilarious, and heartwarming reality of raising tiny humans.

So, take a deep breath. Grab that (probably cold) coffee. And remember—you're not in this alone.
You're an incredible mom. And this journey? It's wild, wonderful, and absolutely worth it.

Now, let's dive in.

Motherhood is a Rollercoaster!

It is full of highs, lows, laughter, and moments that leave you wondering if you're actually losing your mind. This book is here to remind you that you're not alone, you're doing better than you think, and sometimes, the best thing you can do is just laugh through the chaos.

Here's what's waiting for you inside:

Words of Wisdom:

Gentle reminders that perfection isn't the goal—love is. Because spoiler: no one has it all figured out, and that's perfectly okay.

Lighthearted Anecdotes:

Because sometimes, all you can do is laugh—whether it's at the toddler meltdown over the "wrong" color cup or the fact that your child calls you in for an "emergency" just to hand you a toy banana.

Practical Tips:

From handling epic meltdowns to sneaking in self-care without guilt, this book is packed with real-life mom hacks to help you survive and thrive.

Heartfelt Reflections:

The beauty of motherhood isn't in the big moments—it's in the tiny, everyday ones. The sleepy cuddles, the unexpected "I love yous," and the way their little hand still reaches for yours.

A Whole Lot of Reassurance:

This book is like a hug in book form—a reminder that you don't have to be perfect to be an incredible mom.

"Being a mother is learning about strengths you didn't know you had and dealing with fears you didn't know existed."

— **Linda Wooten**

CHAPTER 1:
EMBRACING THE EARLY DAYS

The early days of motherhood are a whirlwind of emotions—

- **Love**
- **Exhaustion**
- **Excitement**
- **Uncertainty**

Those first few weeks and months can feel overwhelming, but they are also some of the most precious moments a mother will ever experience.

A newborn's tiny fingers curling around a mother's hand, the warmth of holding them close, and the quiet moments of bonding in the stillness of the night—these are the experiences that shape the foundation of motherhood.

Though the sleepless nights and endless feedings can be challenging, they are also filled with profound beauty.

Here are some words of wisdom to remind you that you are not alone, that your love is enough, and that every struggle is part of a beautiful journey:

"The days are long, but the years are short."

"There is no way to be a perfect mother, but a million ways to be a good one."

"Sometimes, the strength of motherhood is greater than natural laws."

"Motherhood: All love begins and ends there."

"You are doing better than you think. This moment is hard, but it will pass, and you will look back with pride."

"Babies don't keep. Hold them, love them, and soak in every second."

"A mother's love is endless, her patience immeasurable, and her sacrifices uncountable."

"Your instincts as a mother are stronger than you realize. Trust yourself, and trust your journey."

"You won't remember how tired you were, but you'll remember how small they felt in your arms."

"The days are long, but the years are short."

"There is no way to be a perfect mother, but a million ways to be a good one."

"Sometimes, the strength of motherhood is greater than natural laws."

"Motherhood: All love begins and ends there."

"You are doing better than you think. This moment is hard, but it will pass, and you will look back with pride."

"Babies don't keep. Hold them, love them, and soak in every second."

"A mother's love is endless, her patience immeasurable, and her sacrifices uncountable."

"Your instincts as a mother are stronger than you realize. Trust yourself, and trust your journey."

"You won't remember how tired you were, but you'll remember how small they felt in your arms."

1. The Great Nappy Explosion of 2 am

You know you're officially a mom when you can change a nappy with one hand while half-asleep—until the incident happens.

Picture this: it's 2 AM, your baby has just given you a sweet little smile, and for a brief moment, you think, Wow, I've got this! Then, out of nowhere—BAM! A nappy explosion that defies the laws of physics.

How did it reach the walls?

How is it in your hair?

Some mysteries of motherhood will never be solved.

2. The "Sleep When the Baby Sleeps" Lie

Ah, the classic advice: Just sleep when the baby sleeps! Lovely in theory, completely unrealistic in practice.

Because when the baby finally falls asleep, do you:
a) Do laundry?
b) Take a shower?
c) Stare at them like a creep because they're just so darn cute?
d) Start Googling "why is my baby making weird noises when sleeping?"

Spoiler alert:

You choose d) every time.

3. The One-Armed Mom Life

Once you become a mom, you unlock a hidden superpower: doing everything with one hand.

Cooking? One hand. Brushing your teeth? One hand. Making a cup of tea?

Well, you'll make it, but you won't actually drink it until it's gone cold. Motherhood is just a series of half-finished cups of tea.

4. The "Why Am I Crying?" Phase

One minute, you're fine. The next, you're sobbing over a TV advert featuring a puppy, or because your baby's outgrown their first onesie (even though they only wore it twice).

Motherhood turns you into a walking, talking emotional rollercoaster. And honestly? It's kind of beautiful.

5. The First Outing Disaster

Getting out of the house with a newborn feels like preparing for a week-long expedition. You've packed everything: nappies, wipes, spare clothes, extra spare clothes, bottles, snacks (for you, obviously).

You finally make it to the shops, feeling like a champion—until you realize you've forgotten one crucial thing: the baby bag.

Well, at least you remembered the snacks.

CHAPTER 2:
FINDING BALANCE

As a mother, finding balance can often feel like an impossible task. Between work, home, relationships, and personal well-being, the demands never seem to end.

It's easy to put yourself last while trying to meet everyone else's needs, but balance is not about doing everything perfectly—it's about prioritizing what truly matters.

It's okay to ask for help, to take breaks, and to recognize that you cannot pour from an empty cup.

Self-care is not selfish; it is essential. A well-rested, nurtured mother is better equipped to love, guide, and support her children.

Here are some words of wisdom to help navigate the journey of balance:

"You can do anything, but not everything."

"Balance is not something you find, it's something you create."

"Your worth is not measured by how much you get done in a day."

"Give yourself the same grace and kindness you so freely give to others."

"Some days you will conquer the world. Other days, brushing your hair will be a victory. Both are okay."

"It's okay to step back, slow down, and just breathe."

"Motherhood is not a race to be perfect. It's a journey of love, learning, and showing up the best way you can."

"Some days, balance looks like a clean house and a home-cooked meal. Other days, it looks like survival mode and ordering pizza. Both are valid."

"You are not failing just because you need a break. You are human, and even superheroes need to rest."

"Balance isn't about dividing your time evenly between everything. It's about knowing what needs your heart the most in each moment"

"Motherhood is about finding harmony, not perfection. Some days are messy, some are magical— most are both."

"Taking time for yourself doesn't mean you love your kids any less. It means you want to be the best version of yourself for them"

"It's not about doing it all. It's about doing what matters most in the moment."

"Let go of the guilt. You are doing your best, and that is enough"

"Balance is knowing when to push forward and when to give yourself permission to rest."

Remember, balance is not about perfection. It's about making intentional choices that allow you to care for your family while also honoring yourself. The goal is not to do it all but to do what matters most with love and presence.

1. The Myth of the "Perfect Routine"

Before kids, you probably thought balance meant having a solid daily routine—you know, waking up early, sipping coffee in peace, maybe even squeezing in a little yoga. Then motherhood happened.

Now, "balance" looks like drinking half a cup of cold coffee while holding a baby, answering texts with your toes, and celebrating if you manage to shower before lunchtime.

2. The Laundry Pile That Never Ends

You do a load of laundry, fold it, feel accomplished... and then turn around to see a fresh mountain of baby clothes, bibs, and mysteriously damp burp cloths. You blink twice. Did you even put the baby in this many outfits today?

Scientists may never explain how laundry breeds overnight, but moms everywhere know—it's a real phenomenon.

3. The "Self-Care" Struggle

Every mom is told to "make time for self-care." Sounds great, right?

So, you decide to take a long bath, light some candles, maybe even put on a face mask.

Then—WAAAAHHH! The baby needs you, the toddler is suspiciously quiet, and your relaxing bath turns into a 60-second shower while singing the Peppa Pig theme tune

4. The Grocery Store Sprint

Shopping before kids was a leisurely experience—you'd stroll the aisles, compare brands, maybe browse the seasonal section. Shopping after kids is a military operation. You strategically plan the fastest route, mentally prepare for public tantrums, and attempt to make it to checkout before someone throws a cereal box on the floor. Spoiler alert: you will fail.

5. The "I'll Just Sit for a Second" Trap

Ever tried sitting down when your kid is awake? The second your bum touches the couch, someone needs something. A snack, a toy, help finding that one specific sock.

It's like your children have a radar that detects Mom in Rest Mode—and their mission is to stop it at all costs.

CHAPTER 3: THE POWER OF PATIENCE

Patience is one of the greatest virtues a mother can cultivate.

From sleepless nights and tantrums to the many challenges of growing children, patience becomes the quiet strength that carries a mother through.

It is in the deep breaths, the gentle words, and the understanding that children are learning and growing every day.

There will be moments of frustration, exhaustion, and self-doubt, but patience allows you to respond with love instead of reaction.

It is in these moments that children learn the most—not just from what you say, but from how you model calmness and understanding.

Here are some words of wisdom to remind you of the power of patience:

"Patience is not the ability to wait, but how you act while you're waiting."

"A moment of patience in a moment of anger saves a hundred moments of regret."

"Your child is not giving you a hard time; your child is having a hard time"

"Breathe. This too shall pass.

"Children do not remember how quickly you got things done, but they will remember how kindly you responded"

"Every tough phase is just that—a phase. Keep going."

"Motherhood is teaching without words. Let your patience be the lesson"

"Patience isn't about never feeling frustrated—it's about choosing love even when you do."

"Some of the best lessons are learned in the pauses. Breathe before you react"

"You are growing patience the same way your child is growing—one difficult moment at a time"

"Little hearts take time to understand big emotions. Lead with patience, and they will follow."

"One day, the things that test your patience the most will be the things you miss the most."

"The loudest lessons are taught in silence. A deep breath, a soft word, and a calm presence teach more than any lecture ever could."

"Respond with love even when it's hard—especially when it's hard."

"Your patience today is shaping the way your child will handle life tomorrow."

"Motherhood will test your patience in ways you never imagined, but it will also expand your heart in ways you never thought possible"

"One deep breath can change the course of an entire moment. Pause before you react—you'll never regret it"

"The days you show the most patience are the days you grow the most as a mother."

"Remember, your child is learning how to handle frustration by watching you."

"Grace, deep breaths, and laughter—these are the secrets to surviving the toughest moments."

Patience is a practice, not a perfect skill.

Give yourself grace on the tough days and celebrate the small victories.

With every deep breath, every soft response, and every moment of understanding.

You are shaping a child's heart with love.

1. The Toddler Negotiation Olympics

If you think you're patient, try reasoning with a toddler who insists on wearing a superhero cape, one sock, and absolutely no pants to the supermarket.

You'll spend 20 minutes negotiating, only to realize you've been outsmarted by a three-year-old who now has a lollipop AND no pants. Lesson learned: pick your battles—and always carry emergency trousers.

2. The Slowest. Walk. Ever.

You had big plans to take a quick walk around the block—maybe even get some fresh air and clear your mind. But your toddler has other ideas. Every leaf must be examined. Every rock must be picked up. Every ant must be waved at. A 5-minute walk now takes 45 minutes.

Deep breaths, Mama. The ants are very important.

3. The Bedtime Stalling Masterclass

Bedtime should be simple: bath, book, bed. Instead, it turns into bath, 17 books, water request, another toilet trip, a deep conversation about dinosaurs, an existential crisis, and suddenly your child wants to discuss tomorrow's lunch plans.

You could rush them... but let's be honest—this is just the patience marathon you didn't sign up for.

4. The "I Do It Myself" Phase

There's nothing like the joy of watching your little one learn new things... until they enter the "I do it myself!" stage. Suddenly, putting on shoes takes 15 minutes, buckling their car seat is a 20-minute event, and pouring juice? Prepare for an orange juice tsunami.

You tell yourself to let them be independent, but also... why does getting out the door feel like an Olympic sport?

5. The Mystery of the Never-Ending "Why?"

You thought you had patience... until the "Why?" phase hit.

"Why is the sky blue?"

"Why do birds fly?"

"Why can't I eat cake for breakfast?"

"Why do I have to wear shoes?"

"Why do you look tired, mommy?" (Oh, I don't know, darling... WHY?)

At some point, you just answer "Because I said so" and accept defeat.

CHAPTER 4:
CHERISHING THE LITTLE MOMENTS

In the midst of busy days and endless responsibilities, it's easy to overlook the small, beautiful moments that make motherhood special.

But it is often in these simple, everyday experiences that the greatest joy is found.

Here are some words of wisdom to help you slow down and cherish the little moments:

"One day, you'll long for the fingerprints on the windows, the toys scattered on the floor, and the little voices calling your name. These are the golden days.

The magic of childhood isn't in big events—it's in bedtime stories, belly laughs, and the way they reach for your hand without thinking.

'Your child won't remember the mess, the stress, or the to-do lists. They will remember how loved they felt."

"One day, you'll realize it was never just a bedtime story, never just a hug, never just a moment. It was always more."

"Slow down. The dishes will wait. The laundry will keep. But this moment, right now, is a once-in-a-lifetime memory in the making."

"The days feel long, but the moments pass in an instant. Hold them, love them, and be present."

"Little giggles, messy kisses, sleepy snuggles—these are the things you'll never wish away."

"The best part of motherhood isn't in the milestones, it's in the quiet moments in between."

"You don't have to do anything extraordinary to make childhood magical. Just be there"

"The simplest moments—rocking them to sleep, listening to their stories, holding their tiny hands—will be the ones that stay with you forever."

""One day, they will outgrow your lap, but never your heart."

"Motherhood isn't about keeping up. It's about slowing down enough to notice the moments that matter most."

"Take the picture. Say yes to one more cuddle. Hold them just a little longer. One day, you'll be so glad you did."

Take time to embrace the laughter, the cuddles, the tiny voices calling for you. These are the moments that make motherhood truly meaningful.

1. The 0.2-Second Cuddle

You dream of those heartwarming, movie-worthy cuddles where your child snuggles into your chest, sighs contentedly, and whispers, "I love you, mommy." Reality? You get a 0.2-second side hug before they wriggle away, yelling, "Let go, Mom! I have things to do!" Well, at least you tried.

2. The "Mom, Watch This!" Marathon

Nothing says cherishing the moment like watching your child do the same "cool trick" 57 times in a row.

"Mom, watch this!"

"Mom, did you see that?"

"Wait, Mom, I'm gonna do it again—WATCH!"

Spoiler: It's the same jump off the sofa every time. But you cheer like it's the Olympics because, well, that's motherhood.

3. The First Time They Copy You (Oops!)

You try to be a good role model. You really do. But then one day, you stub your toe, mutter ahem a "grown-up" word, and suddenly your toddler is walking around the house dropping mini F-bombs like it's their new favorite word. Nothing makes you cherish your influence more than hearing your own sass repeated with perfect accuracy.

4. The Masterpiece That Must Be Admired

Your child draws a beautiful picture... well, beautiful in a modern art kind of way. You squint at it: Is that a dog? A potato? An alien? Doesn't matter—you act THRILLED and immediately put it on the fridge like it belongs in the Louvre.

Because one day, they'll stop handing you their doodles, and you'll actually miss your fridge looking like an abstract art gallery.

5. The Midnight "I Love You"

After a long, exhausting day of tantrums, mess, and 47 snack requests, you finally collapse into bed. Then, in the middle of the night, a tiny voice whispers, "mommy?" You brace yourself for another request... but instead, they simply say, "I love you."

And just like that, every hard moment melts away

CHAPTER 5:
RAISING RESILIENT CHILDREN

Raising resilient children means teaching them confidence, independence, and strength.

It's about allowing them to make mistakes, supporting them through challenges, and empowering them to believe in themselves.

Resilience isn't about avoiding hardship; it's about learning how to navigate it with courage and perseverance.

Here are some words of wisdom to guide you in fostering resilience in your children:

"Children need the freedom to fail so they can learn how to succeed."

"Every challenge your child faces is an opportunity to teach them strength."

"Teach them to stand tall, even when the world feels heavy."

"Resilience is not about never falling, but about always getting back up."

"A confident child is one who knows they are loved unconditionally, even when they make mistakes."

Let them struggle a little; it's how they grow strong.

Your words become their inner voice. Choose them wisely.

Children don't need perfection. They need to see how to handle imperfection with grace.

The most important thing you can give your child is belief in their own ability.

Building resilience takes time, patience, and encouragement. It means allowing your child to take risks, make mistakes, and learn from them. It's about showing them that failure isn't the opposite of success—it's part of the journey toward it. By raising resilient children, you are giving them one of life's greatest gifts: the ability to face the world with confidence and strength.

1. The "I'm fine!" Phenomenon

Your child will trip over thin air, face-plant onto the floor, and pop back up like nothing happened. Meanwhile, you are having a mini heart attack, rushing over with the first-aid kit.

"Are you okay?!"

Shrugs "I'm fine."

"Are you sure?"

"Yeah, but can I have ice cream now?"

Apparently, kids bounce better than logic.

2. The Battle of the Broccoli

Nothing builds resilience like trying to get a child to eat vegetables. You've tried everything—hiding it in pasta, calling it a "superhero snack," even pretending broccoli gives them magical powers. Still, they stare at it like you've put radioactive waste on their plate.

Then, two days later, you catch them eating a random leaf off the floor like it's no big deal.

3. The Shoe-on-the-Wrong-Foot Confidence

Your child insists on dressing themselves—great!

Except their shoes are always on the wrong feet. You gently point it out, and they stare at you with unwavering confidence and say, "No, they're perfect."

So now you have a child walking around looking like a tiny, determined penguin.

And honestly? Respect.

4. The "I Can Do It Myself" Disaster

One day, they insist on pouring their own cereal.

You brace yourself.

You hold your breath.

You watch as an entire box of Cheerios spills all over the floor.

Instead of admitting defeat, they cheerfully eat the ones closest to the bowl like nothing happened. Resilience in action.

5. The Toddler Comeback Game

Kids have an unbelievable ability to bounce back—not just from falls, but from full-blown emotional meltdowns.

One second: screaming because you cut their sandwich the wrong way.

The next second: laughing hysterically at a fart noise.

Meanwhile, you're still emotionally recovering from the sandwich crisis.

CHAPTER 6:
SELF-CARE IS NOT SELFISH

As a mother, it's easy to pour every ounce of energy into your family while leaving little for yourself.

But self-care is not a luxury—it's a necessity. Taking time to nurture your own well-being allows you to be the best version of yourself for your children.

When you care for yourself, you model self-respect, balance, and emotional health for your family.

Here are some empowering words to remind you of the importance of self-care:

"You can't pour from an empty cup. Take care of yourself first."

"Self-care is not indulgence; it is self-preservation."

"Taking time for yourself isn't selfish. It's essential."

"A well-rested, happy mother is a better mother."

"Give yourself permission to rest. You are doing enough."

"Taking care of yourself means your children get the best of you, not what's left of you."

"You are allowed to take up space, to say no, and to prioritize yourself."

"Self-care is how you take your power back."

Taking time for yourself is not about neglecting your family—it's about ensuring that you have the energy, patience, and strength to give them your best.

You deserve care just as much as anyone else. Prioritize your well-being, and watch how it positively impacts both you and your family.

1. The "Relaxing" Bath Fantasy vs. Reality

Before kids, self-care meant long, luxurious baths, candles, and a good book. After kids? You attempt a bath, but within two minutes:

Someone bursts in needing a snack.

Another one starts crying about absolutely nothing.

A plastic dinosaur mysteriously appears in the water.

You hear crash noises and now you're stressed instead of relaxed.

So, you settle for a 30-second rinse and pretend it was spa-like.

2. The Coffee That Never Gets Drunk Hot

Once upon a time, you drank coffee while it was hot. Now?

You make the coffee.

The baby cries.

You reheat the coffee.

Someone needs help finding their shoes.

You reheat the coffee again.

It's now 4 PM and you're still sipping lukewarm disappointment.

3. The "Quick Nap" Illusion

You finally get five minutes to rest, so you close your eyes. Just as you drift off...

MOMMMMM!!!

CRASH!

Someone's standing 2 inches from your face whispering,

"Are you awake?"

Yes, darling. I am now.

4. The Solo Trip to the Supermarket = A Mini Holiday

Self-care doesn't have to be fancy. Sometimes, grocery shopping alone is a luxury retreat.

No one is asking for snacks.

No one is throwing things into the trolley.

You can actually walk at a normal human pace.

You even consider taking the long way home, just for the silence.

5. The Guilt-Free Snack Stash

You tell your kids to share, but when it comes to your secret stash of chocolate, that's a solo treat.

You hide in the pantry.

You chew as quietly as humanly possible.

You deny everything when they ask, "What's in your mouth, Mom?"

Self-care, ladies. It's survival.

CHAPTER 7:
BUILDING A SUPPORT SYSTEM

Motherhood is a beautiful journey, but it is not meant to be walked alone. Having a strong support system—whether it's family, friends, or a community—can make all the difference.

Leaning on others, sharing experiences, and seeking guidance not only lightens the load but also brings joy and reassurance in times of struggle.

Here are some words of wisdom on the power of a support system:

"It takes a village to raise a child, but it also takes a village to support a mother."

"Surround yourself with those who lift you up, not those who wear you down."

"Asking for help is not a sign of weakness, but of wisdom."

"A mother's strength is limitless, but even the strongest need a hand to hold"

"You were never meant to do this alone. Seek support, embrace connection"

"True friends don't just celebrate your joys; they stand beside you in your struggles."

"Strong mothers build strong communities. Together, we rise."

"You are not failing if you ask for help. You are being human."

Building a support system is about finding people who understand, encourage, and uplift you.

Whether through family, friendships, mom groups, or online communities, know that you are never alone. Reach out, connect, and embrace the power of togetherness.

1. The "Texting Mom Friends at 2 AM" Club

You know you've found your people when you can text another mom at 2 AM like:

"Is it normal for a baby to grunt in their sleep like an old man?"

"Why won't my toddler wear trousers? Is this a phase or a personality trait?"

"How do I make my child eat something other than beige food?"

No "hey, how are you?"—just straight to panic mode. And the best part? They answer.

2. The Group Chat Lifeline

Having a solid mom group chat means:

Sharing horror stories of public toddler meltdowns.

Sending memes about needing a holiday from your children.

Trading hacks on how to sneak vegetables into food (even though everyone secretly just gives up and serves pasta).

Honestly, this chat is more important than most of your actual responsibilities.

3. The Partner "Help" That's Not Really Help

You: "Can you watch the baby while I shower?"

Him: "Yeah, of course!"

Reality: You come out of the shower to find the baby still in a nappy from three hours ago, toys everywhere, and your partner asleep on the sofa.

So now, instead of feeling refreshed, you're MORE stressed than before. Classic.

4. The Babysitting Negotiations

Asking a relative to babysit is like delicate diplomacy.

"Hey Mom, what are you up to this Saturday?"

"Oh, nothing much..."

"GREAT! Because we were thinking—"

"No. Not happening. Last time they smeared yogurt on my dog."

Fair enough

5. The "You Too?!" Friendships

You know you've met a mom soulmate when you both admit:

You've let your kid watch Peppa Pig for an hour just for some peace.

You also pretend not to hear "Muuuum" sometimes.

Your idea of a wild night is being in bed by 9:30 PM.

There's nothing better than realizing you're not the only one just winging it.

CHAPTER 8:
LESSONS FROM OUR MOTHERS

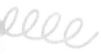

The wisdom of our mothers and grandmothers is a priceless gift passed down through generations. Their experiences, sacrifices, and love have shaped us into the women and mothers we are today. By reflecting on their words and actions, we gain insight into the timeless lessons that guide us in raising our own children.

Here are some reflections on the wisdom of mothers:

"A mother's love is the foundation on which we build our lives."

"The lessons our mothers teach us never fade; they echo in our hearts forever"

"Strength, patience, and kindness—these are the gifts our mothers pass down to us"

"Mothers may not always have the right words, but their love speaks volumes."

"The best parenting advice often comes from the women who raised us."

"Our mothers showed us what it means to love unconditionally. Now, we do the same for our children."

"A mother's wisdom is timeless—it lives on in the hearts of her children and grandchildren."

Learning from the past helps us navigate the present and prepare for the future.

Whether through their words, their actions, or their unwavering love, our mothers have left us with a blueprint for raising our own children with grace, resilience, and warmth.

Cherish their lessons, honor their sacrifices, and pass their wisdom forward.

1. "Because I Said So" is a Legitimate Answer

Growing up, you swore you'd never use your mom's favorite response: "Because I said so."

Fast forward to today, and here you are, staring at your child who's asking, "But why can't I bring my pet rock to the supermarket?"

You take a deep breath... and it happens. "Because I said so."

And just like that, you have become your mother.

2. The Magic of Mom's Spit

As a child, nothing was more horrifying than your mom licking her thumb and wiping your face in public. Disgusting!

Then one day, you notice your child has mystery food stuck to their cheek, and without thinking, you lick your thumb and wipe it off.

Your transformation is complete.

3. The "One Day You'll Understand" Prophecy

Mom used to say, "One day, you'll understand."

You rolled your eyes.

Then, motherhood hit.

And suddenly, you understand everything.

Why she sighed deeply before answering "Muuuum?" for the 50th time.

Why she was always eating the "broken biscuits."

Why she told you to "enjoy sleep while you can."

Mom, I get it now. I'm sorry for everything.

4. The "Don't Waste Food" Guilt Trip

Your mom never let food go to waste.

"There are starving children who would love that broccoli."
"You're not leaving this table until your plate is empty."

Now? You find yourself saying the exact same thing—except your kid still refuses to eat anything green.

Meanwhile, you're standing in the kitchen, eating their cold leftovers straight off the plate, because mom guilt won't let you throw it away.

5. The Mysterious Mom Powers

Your mom always knew everything.

Who broke the vase? She knew.

Who ate the last biscuit? She knew.

Where your missing shoe was? She knew.

Now, you have the same powers.

You know when your child is lying.

You know the exact moment they're about to cause chaos.
You can sense silence from another room (and know it means trouble).

Mom intuition is real. Use it wisely.

CHAPTER 9:
OVERCOMING MOM GUILT

Mom guilt is something nearly every mother experiences at some point.

The pressure to be perfect, to always be present, and to do everything "right" can be overwhelming. But perfection is an impossible standard.

The truth is, being a great mom isn't about doing everything flawlessly—it's about showing up with love, authenticity, and a willingness to grow.

Here are some words of encouragement to help let go of guilt and embrace authenticity:

There is no perfect mother, only real ones.

"You are doing better than you think. Your love is enough."

"Your child doesn't need perfection; they just need you."

"Let go of the guilt. Embrace the joy."

"A happy, fulfilled mother raises happy, fulfilled children"

"Every mother struggles. You are not alone."

"The fact that you worry about being a good mom means that you already are one"

Releasing mom guilt starts with recognizing that you are enough just as you are.

Your love, effort, and presence matter more than any unattainable standard.

Embrace the imperfections, celebrate the wins, and trust that you are exactly the mother your child needs.

1. The "Healthy Lunch" Guilt Trip

You start the week strong: freshly cut fruit, homemade sandwiches, organic snacks.

By Wednesday? Crackers and cheese.

By Friday? A packet of biscuits and a strong hope that the school serves actual food.

Cue mom guilt—but hey, they ate, didn't they?

2. The "Screen Time Spiral"

You tell yourself: "No screens today!"

8 AM: We're doing crafts, this is amazing!

10 AM: Okay, 15 minutes of TV while I clean up.

2 PM: Maybe a little more so I can drink my coffee.

5 PM: They've now watched 4 hours of Peppa Pig, and I don't even care.

Mom guilt kicks in, but honestly, you needed the break.

3. The Forgotten "mommy, Watch This!"

Your child yells, "mommy, watch this!" 57 times.

You watch the first 10.

You pretend to watch the next 20.

You completely zone out around #45.

Suddenly, "mommy! You weren't looking!"

Now, you're apologizing like you missed their Olympic debut instead of the same jump they've done for the last hour.

4. The "I Snuck Chocolate" Betrayal

You tell your kids they can't have sugar before bed.

Then, the second they're asleep, you sneak into the kitchen for a secret chocolate feast.

But just as you take that first glorious bite—

"mommy, what are you eating?"

Busted. Now, you either share or lie. (Hint: You lie. It's "mommy medicine.")

5. The "Left My Kid at School" Horror

You're 5 minutes late to school pickup, and you already feel like the worst mom ever.

Your child greets you with: "mommy, I thought you forgot me forever."

Five minutes. That's all it took for them to act like you abandoned them in the wilderness.

Mom guilt level: MAXIMUM.

CHAPTER 10:
CELEBRATING MILESTONES

Every milestone—big or small—is a reminder of how far both you and your child have come.

Whether it's a first step, a graduation, or a birthday, these moments deserve to be cherished and celebrated.

Milestones are not just about achievements; they are about growth, perseverance, and the love that has guided the journey.

Here are some words to celebrate these special moments:

Here are some words to celebrate these special moments:
"Every milestone is a chapter in your child's story—celebrate each page.

The days are long, but the years are short. Savor every moment

Every little achievement is a step towards a bright future.

You are not just raising a child; you are raising a future.

"Behind every proud moment is a mother who believed."

"From first words to first steps, every milestone is a testament to love."

"These are the moments you'll look back on and cherish forever."

"Your child's milestones are yours too—celebrate the journey."

Life moves quickly, and these moments pass in the blink of an eye. Take the time to celebrate, reflect, and embrace each step of your child's journey.

These milestones are proof of love, effort, and the beautiful bond you share.

1. The First Steps... That You Missed

You've been waiting for months for your baby to take their first steps. Camera ready, eyes locked in, cheering them on.

Then, one day, you step out for 30 seconds to pee... and BAM! They take their first steps while staring at the dog.

You rush back, begging them to do it again—but nope. They've retired from walking for the day.

Cue the mom guilt and a deep sigh as you accept that the dog got the VIP moment, not you.

2. The "I Wasn't Ready" Kindergarten Drop-Off

You spend years dreaming about the day your little one starts school, imagining tears, hugs, and dramatic goodbyes. Instead, you get:

"Bye, Mom!" (runs off without looking back)

You, standing there, ready to cry—but now wondering if you should be offended.

Now, you're the only emotional one while they've fully moved on in under five seconds. Rude.

3. The Birthday Party Chaos

You promise yourself this year will be a simple celebration.

Then, before you know it:

There's a balloon arch in your living room.

You've spent three days making a themed cake that your child takes one bite of.

The kids have eaten too much sugar and are now parkour-ing off the furniture.

By the end, you're exhausted, and your child's favorite part?

The £2 party bag toy. Of course.

4. The Potty Training "Oops"

You finally get your toddler to use the potty—a huge milestone! You celebrate, do a little dance, and feel like a champion.

Then, the next day, you proudly let them wear big kid underwear at the shops.

...Big mistake. BIG mistake.

You learn two things that day:

Always carry spare clothes.

Your child has zero shame about announcing, "mommy, I just did a wee right here!" in the middle of the supermarket.

5. The First Tooth Fairy Fail

Your child loses their first tooth. It's magical, exciting... and you totally forget to swap the tooth for money.

The next morning:

"mommy, the Tooth Fairy forgot me!"

You, still half-asleep: "Uh... maybe she got stuck in traffic?"

Cue the panic as you scramble for a coin and casually "find" it under the pillow, claiming it was there the whole time! Crisis (barely) averted.

HEARTFELT REFLECTIONS

Motherhood is a journey made up of tiny, fleeting moments—the ones that catch you off guard, stop you in your tracks, and make you realize, this is it. This is the good stuff.

It's not the big milestones that truly define motherhood. It's the little in-between moments—the ones that slip by too fast, the ones we wish we could bottle up and keep forever.

1. The Sleepy Midnight Cuddles

There's something about holding your baby in the middle of the night, when the world is quiet and it's just the two of you. Yes, you're exhausted. Yes, you'd do anything for just one solid night of sleep. But in that moment, as their tiny hand rests against your chest, their breath soft and steady, you realize this is temporary. One day, they won't need you in the middle of the night. And suddenly, you don't mind being awake so much.

2. The "I Love You, mommy" Out of Nowhere

You could be in the middle of the school run chaos, trying to find missing shoes, rushing out the door, mentally making a list of everything you forgot—when suddenly, your child looks up at you and says, "I love you, mommy."

No reason, no prompting. Just pure, heart-melting love. And for a second, everything else fades away.

3. The Tiny Hand in Yours

One day, your child will stop reaching for your hand. But for now, their little fingers find yours instinctively—at the supermarket, crossing the road, or just walking through the house. That small hand in yours is a reminder: you are their safe place.

And when they let go without thinking one day, you'll realize how much you miss the weight of that tiny hand in your palm.

4. The Uncontrollable Laughter

There are moments in motherhood when the laughter is so pure, so ridiculous, so out of control that you can't help but join in. Maybe it's your toddler mispronouncing a word in the funniest way. Maybe it's your child putting underwear on their head and calling it a hat. Or maybe it's just the sheer delirium of being so overtired that everything is suddenly hilarious.

Motherhood teaches you to laugh more, worry less, and embrace the chaos.

5. The Way They Look at You

Even on the days when you feel like you're failing—when the house is a mess, when patience is running thin, when you wonder if you're doing anything right—your child still looks at you like you're the best person in the world.

To them, you are comfort. You are safety. You are love.

And that's when it hits you: you don't have to be perfect. You just have to be theirs.

Motherhood isn't about having it all together. It's about loving fiercely, embracing the mess, and cherishing the little moments—because one day, these moments will be the ones you miss the most.

So, hold them close. Laugh with them often. And know that even on the hard days, you are everything they need.

PRACTICAL TIPS

Motherhood is a beautiful journey, but let's be real—it's also a full-contact sport. Some days feel like winning an Olympic medal in patience; other days, you're hiding in the bathroom eating chocolate. Here's a mix of survival tips, wisdom, and good old-fashioned mom hacks to keep you going.

1. Handling Meltdowns Like a Pro

The Supermarket Showdown
You're in the middle of the supermarket, holding a loaf of bread, when suddenly your child throws themselves on the floor like a footballer faking an injury. A full-blown, screaming, limbs flailing, red-faced tantrum.

Mom Hack:
The Whisper Technique – Instead of raising your voice, whisper. It freaks them out just enough to pause.

"Wow, you're really going for the Oscar, huh? Want to try again, or should we call Hollywood?"

The Distraction Method – Suddenly point at nothing and gasp, "Oh my gosh! Did you see that?!" Works 60% of the time.

If all else fails, throw them over your shoulder like a sack of potatoes and leave with dignity.

2. Sneaking in Self-Care Without the Guilt

The "Luxury" Shower Experience
Taking a shower should be simple, but somehow, it feels like a heist movie.

Mom Hack:
Shower when they nap? Nope, because that's your snack-eating, phone-scrolling time.

Shower with the door open? Risky, but better than hearing "Muuuum!" 47 times.

Shower at night? Peaceful, but then you're too tired to enjoy it.

Solution? "mommy's Spa Time" – Hand them a snack, turn on a cartoon, and enjoy five whole minutes of uninterrupted bliss.

3. The Art of Hiding Snacks
You deserve that chocolate, but eating it in front of your kids means they'll immediately want some.

Mom Hack:
The Classic Pantry Hideout – Eat behind a cupboard door like a sugar-addicted ninja.

The Fake Healthy Snack Trick – Put your sweets in a bag labeled "Kale Chips". They won't touch it.

The Bathroom Escape – Lock the door and pretend you're "using the toilet." (You're actually eating cookies in peace.)

4. Mastering the 30-Second Nap

Your toddler refuses to nap, but you need sleep.

Mom Hack:

The "Let's Play a Game" Trick – Tell your kid, "Let's play Sleeping Lions! Whoever moves first loses!" Then close your eyes and pretend it's a nap.

The "I'm Just Resting My Eyes" Move – Lie down on the sofa and let them poke your face every five minutes while you recharge just enough to survive.

If all else fails, coffee and adrenaline will carry you through.

5. Getting Stuff Done Without Losing Your Mind

Cleaning With Kids in the House (Impossible, But We Try)
Trying to clean while kids are awake is like brushing your teeth while eating Oreos.

Mom Hack:

The "Cleaning is a Game" Trick – "Who can put away the most toys in one minute? GO!" (This works exactly twice before they catch on.)

The "Mom Needs Help" Guilt Trip – "mommy is soooo tired, I wish someone would help..." They might pick up one toy.

Or, just accept the mess. A tidy house is a myth created by people without children.

6. The "Getting Out the Door" Struggle

Leaving the house with kids is a military operation.

Mom Hack:

Get Ready in Reverse – Shoes first. Then coats. Then last-minute nappy changes, water bottles, snacks, etc.

The "Bye, I'm Leaving Without You" Trick – Pretend to leave and watch them run to the door in sheer panic.
No matter what, you will still be 20 minutes late. Accept it.

7. Pretending to Know What You're Doing

Your child asks you random, impossible questions like:

"mommy, why is the moon following us?"

"Do fish have friends?"

"Why don't giraffes get dizzy?"

Mom Hack:

Confidently make something up. "Oh, the moon is checking on us to make sure we get home safe."

Google quickly and pretend you always knew.

Throw the question back at them. "Hmm, what do YOU think?" (Buys you time to sip your coffee.)

'Finally motherhood is messy, unpredictable, and sometimes downright hilarious. You won't always get it right, and that's totally okay.
So, laugh through the chaos, sneak in your self-care where you can, and remember: you're doing better than you think!